UNMASKED:

The Science that Suggests Your Muzzle Spreads COVID

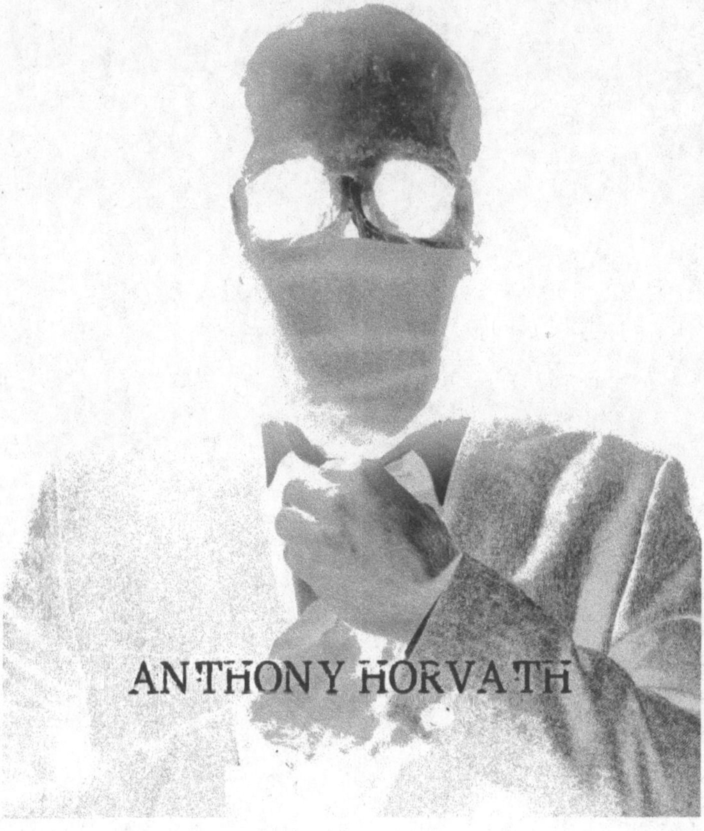

ANTHONY HORVATH

UnMasked

The Science

That Suggests

Your Muzzle Spreads COVID

By

Anthony Horvath

UnMasked: The Science That Suggests Your Muzzle Spreads COVID

By Anthony Horvath

ISBN: 978-1-64594-53-1

Also available in hard cover:
ISBN: 978-1-64594-052-4

V. 12/8/2020

About the Author:

Anthony Horvath has a terminal degree in a field touching on the subject of epistemology. Epistemology can be thought of as 'the study of what we know, why we think we know it, and how certain are we of our knowledge.' This being the case, he adamantly opposes arguments from authority, since they are logical fallacies: something isn't true *just because* an authority asserts it to be true. Therefore, the above information is given reluctantly, as the last thing that the author wants is for anyone to believe what follows *only* because he asserts it. Nonetheless, there is an appropriate role for 'expertise' in the epistemological process, not as an assurance of truth, but at least as an indicator of seriousness. You need no advanced degrees to process what follows. You need only be literate, courageous enough to consider and even, if the evidence supports it, willing to adopt contrarian views, and be ready and able to apply common sense and basic 'laws' of logic. Good luck. If you are in one of the truly vulnerable groups, your life literally could depend on the findings included in this document.

Introduction

It may surprise readers that at the beginning of this whole thing, I supported wearing masks. Indeed, I expressed great irritation that our elites and the complicit media were telling people not to wear masks. I argued vigorously with people who insisted that "masks don't work." In fact, I'm not against wearing masks at all, *per se*. It is the compulsory element, especially as the same arguments and principles used to justify compulsory masking can—and will—be used to justify almost everything else. Does this mean I had a change of heart?

No.

The context matters. Back in February and March of 2020, we could legitimately say we didn't know enough about the novel coronavirus to say with confidence we knew what we were up against. It was in the context of a disease with (still) suspicious connections to a Chinese bioweapons lab. It was in the context of… wait for it… "fifteen days to slow the spread." (ikr; you can stop laughing now!) And, it must be made absolutely clear, when I supported wearing masks, it was with the expectation we would use masks that *were actually effective*. Crazy, right?

At the time, it never crossed my mind that anyone would seriously consider cloth masks to be sufficient. Tradesmen, like painters, don't go to the big box store and buy cloth masks to protect them from dust and fumes. Firefighters, when obtaining their hazmat certifications, are not told the appropriate PPE for responding to a biohazard incident is a cloth mask, nor even a surgical mask, nor even *only* N95s![1] That is to say, in the real world, long before politics and agendas intervened, no one was silly enough to think that a cloth mask would accomplish anything.

So, my advocacy for masks importantly was for masks that would work. That's a far cry from where we are today, as I will demonstrate in this essay.

Connected to this is the awareness that masks had limited value in narrowly constrained situations (eg, like a painter while he

---

[1] As argued in what follows, in the real world it is acknowledged that the eyes and skin in general are vulnerable to biological contamination. Thus, goggles, hoods, full body gowns, and so on are urged, which meet NFPA 1999 standards, which in turn require tests for bio-penetration. For an example of what they might wear—in the real world—visit: https://www.kappler.com/l100

In the real world, your local firefighter is probably not going to have the appropriate gear and will set the perimeter until those who do have them, arrive. But don't worry, I'm sure your cloth mask will protect you!

is painting), which, if the plan is to "slow the spread" (please, it would help if you wouldn't laugh so obnoxiously whenever I bring that up) maybe, just maybe, masks that work would, in fact, slow the spread (stop laughing), providing our health care system and researchers a chance to ramp up their own response.

Anyone with two brain cells to rub together now knows that the "slow the spread" scheme was an outright lie. No doubt, there were many people who sincerely thought that was our genuine strategy, and many of these were willing to abide by the various mandates, such as stay at home orders, with the understanding that no one really believes we can fully stop a highly transmissible virus from transmitting. The scheme quickly morphed into a completely unrealistic goal having nothing to do with allowing our health care system to keep up, and instead aimed to prevent the spread of ALL cases altogether.

Here again context matters. If we were talking about something as lethal as Ebola, then by all means, additional measures are in order. But, almost eight months in, we know that COVID is very survivable. So survivable, that most 'cases' are asymptomatic. So many, in fact, that we are only discovering them at all because of all of the (mostly unnecessary) testing. You are required, for example, to get a COVID test in order to get a procedure at a clinic, even though you feel perfectly well, and from a clinical point of view, do not have COVID. The PCR tests, which amplify and magnify small traces of the disease are treated as positive results, even if there is virtually zero chance the person testing positive will be transmitting the extremely weakened virus lurking in their bodies.

Masks (that work) to 'slow the spread' against a novel virus? Ok. Masks (that don't work) to perform a national and international full eradication of a no longer novel virus? No. In fact, as I argue in what follows, there is not only very little evidence to suggest that masks of any sort will work ***for that context***, the evidence presently suggests what many of us are actually witnessing: *these measures are actually spreading the virus even more than if we weren't wearing masks at all.*

You will no doubt detect in what follows a certain contempt for the position of "We Need to all Wear Masks (that don't work) to Eradicate Viruses." I tried to scale back that contempt as much as I could, but to be perfectly frank, at this point I'm long past the point where I believe that people of that position can be reasoned with, and what they really need to know is that I, and millions like me, HAVE RUN OUT OF PATIENCE WITH THEM. They need to know this, and I communicate it via my tone, which, I swear, I actually softened up considerably as I edited the document.

What is my (our) problem with them?

It isn't just their irrational and scientifically meritless position. It's their moral smugness and utter certainty that A., people who disagree with them are the worst vermin ever to have walked the earth and B., their willingness—no, eagerness—to attribute any spread of the virus to people 'not complying' rather than consider the possibility that it is the compliance *itself* that is spreading the virus. But there is a C.

C., It is literally the same people who argued with me back in March, telling me NOT to buy or use masks, who are now pompously telling me we absolutely MUST wear masks, or else, Hitler, or something like that.

Not the same *kind* of people. THE EXACT SAME PEOPLE.

Why? What reason do they give? Because the 'experts' say so, that's why! Yes, that's right. In March, the experts said X, and they accepted the proclamation wholesale and argued not on the basis of evidence, but (logical fallacy alert) on the basis of the authority of experts, who continue to argue only on the basis of the authority of experts, rather than on evidence.

You can't reason with people who know nothing of the evidence and don't even care, anyway. You can't argue with people who don't see a disconnect between "fifteen days to slow the spread" and "fifteen months to end death forever!" (or sumthin like that, the goalposts move frequently). You can't argue with people who believe that people in May protesting vigorously about the loss of their livelihoods along with their liberties are bad, bad, bad, people, but then are perfectly fine with people burning down whole city blocks, shoulder to shoulder.

But I didn't write this essay for THEM.

I wrote this essay for those who have noticed that the people getting COVID that they have observed in their own experiences are people who are dutifully complying with every measure thrown at them. "How can this be?" They wonder. I wrote this essay for those who have noticed a very strange thing: in all the places where harsh measures were in place, the virus is nonetheless SURGING.

"How can this be?" I wrote this essay for people who are in known risk groups—people who are age 60 and up, maybe, with co-morbidities, and so on. That is, people who genuinely are at risk and genuinely want to protect themselves. If you want to die, continue to listen to the compulsory mask crowd uncritically. If you want to live, listen to me. Which means, first and foremost, thinking critically and thinking independently, because there are good reasons for believing that our universal masking pretty much ensures the virus spreads, and if you don't want it, then you had better take that into account.

Without further ado, let's get into it.

(Just a heads up, I have also appended a postscript which some will find to be entertaining to read.)

Reminder:

Fair use is invoked for all citations from studies, excerpts, or images made by the WHO, etc.

How can this be? I wrote this essay for people who are in known risk groups—people who are aged and/or suffer with co-morbidities, and so on. That is, people who genuinely are at risk and genuinely want to protect themselves. If you want to die, continue to listen to the compulsory mask crowd uncritically. If you want to live, listen to me. Which means, first and foremost, thinking critically and thinking independently, because there are good reasons for believing that our universal masking policy much ensures the virus spreads and if you don't want it, then you had better take that into account.

Without further ado, let's get into it.

(Just a heads up: I have also appended a postscript which some will find to be entertaining to read.)

Reminder:

Fair use is invoked for all citations from studies, excerpts, or images made by the WHO, etc.

The Evidence Suggests Universal Masking *INCREASES* the Spread of COVID-19

Have you noticed yet that the people most likely to get COVID are those religiously complying with all masking mandates and social distancing to the extreme? I am aware of about a half dozen such cases and I bet more and more people are going to start noticing it as well. Moreover, cases are increasing in all the places where mandates are the strictest and compliance is the highest.

Why would this be happening?

Am I being too subtle? Let's put it more bluntly: it is entirely plausible, if not likely, that wearing masks *demonstrably* spreads COVID; compelling people to wear masks ensures that *more* people get COVID than if they weren't wearing masks at all. This isn't a conspiracy. It is supported by the 'science,' but more and more people don't need the 'science,' as their daily lives fill up with anecdotes of people complying with every mandate thrown at them, nonetheless getting sick.

The assertion that cases are going up in the face of widespread compliance is not anecdote. Studies have been showing it. For example, a recent Marquette University study discovered that the mask-wearing compliance is around 90% in Wisconsin… at the very same time when cases are/were 'surging.'

Examples of this will multiply, and more are given later in the essay. Before we get to that, let's start with showing how what we already know, *from the evidence*, explains or even predicts such paradoxical results.

In a 2010 Oxford study titled "Simple Respiratory Protection—Evaluation of the Filtration Performance of Cloth Masks and Common Fabric Materials Against 20-1000nm Size particles" they assert…

> "… common fabric materials … were tested for … aerosols (20-1000nm) at two different face velocities … and compared with the penetration levels for N95 respirator filter media. The results showed that cloth masks and other fabric materials tested in the study had **40-90% instantaneous penetration levels**…"

Read that last sentence again. Let your eyes hover on that word 'instantaneous' a little longer.

Their summary concludes with:

> "Results obtained in the study show that common fabric materials **may** provide **marginal** protection against nanoparticles including those in the size ranges of virus-containing particles in exhaled breath."

Why should wearing cloth masks that are 40-90% ineffective actually be spreading COVID? This is a different question which we will take up shortly, but the authors of this study set the table for us. They note:

> "These household materials are not designed for respiratory protection **and their use may provide a false sense of protection** because their effectiveness against larger and <1000 nm size particles including viruses is not well understood. This indicates that further studies are needed…"

Emphasis added.

Here, then, are the two most obvious elements which you did not in fact need 'science' to tell you: 1., **cloth** masks are not going to be effective and 2., if you think they are, its going to create 'a false sense of protection.' With that 'false sense of protection,' people who think they are protected will act as though they are protected, but since in fact they are not protected, they will… wait for it… most likely make themselves sick, make others sick, and overwhelm the health care system, endangering first responders, and so on and so forth. You know, the very thing they *say* they are trying to prevent!

The truth about the efficacy of masks, or lack thereof, is no secret. It is evidence such as described above that led the SURGEON GENERAL of the United States to 'tweet' back in February of 2020:

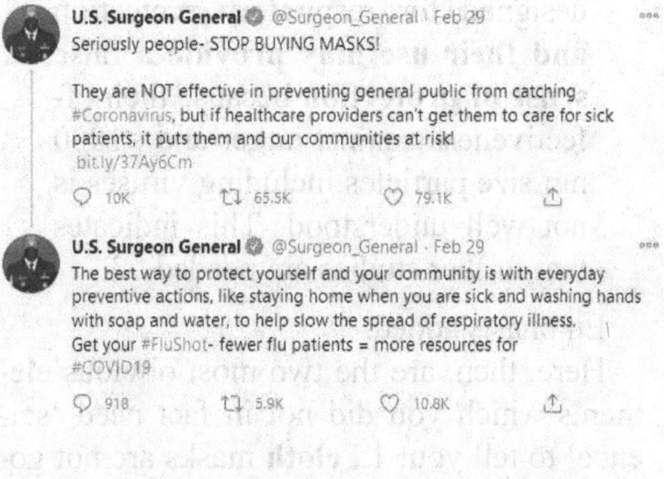

U.S. Surgeon General @Surgeon_General · Feb 29
Seriously people- STOP BUYING MASKS!

They are NOT effective in preventing general public from catching #Coronavirus, but if healthcare providers can't get them to care for sick patients, it puts them and our communities at risk!
bit.ly/37Ay6Cm

10K 65.5K 79.1K

U.S. Surgeon General @Surgeon_General · Feb 29
The best way to protect yourself and your community is with everyday preventive actions, like staying home when you are sick and washing hands with soap and water, to help slow the spread of respiratory illness.
Get your #FluShot- fewer flu patients = more resources for #COVID19

918 5.9K 10.8K

In regards to masks, he was not lying. He was in fact in line with what the 'science' at the time supported. Not long after this, the calls for compulsory muzzling began, and many scientists began raising alarm, because they knew that the studies already in hand not only demonstrated that such measures, in the general population, had little to no empirical basis, but could actually be harmful.

For example, in April of 2020, two scientists, in a commentary which summarized *all the available data* to that point, summed up their conclusions in the very title of their article: "Masks-for-all for COVID-19 not based on sound data." In this article, they observed this about the efficacy of cloth masks:

> "These studies demonstrate that cloth or homemade masks will have very low filter efficiency (2% to 38%)."

What do you call a COVID positive person wearing a mask with only 2% effectiveness coming in contact with a COVID negative person also wearing a mask with only 2% effectiveness? Two Covid positive people. That's what you call them.

Importantly, they continue on to point out that *medical masks* are only nominally better…

> "studies have found a wide range of filter efficiency (2% to 98%), with

most exhibiting 30% to 50% efficiency."

They provide 7 sources to back up this assertion. An effectiveness for *both* cloth and surgical masks as low as 2%, folks. TWO PERCENT. You can't just slap something on your face, even if it is a 'surgical mask,' and think it will 'work.' There are many, many variables involved (hence the wide ranges), not the least of which is understanding that there are different levels of quality in the materials used for all of these masks.

This whole idea that if everyone wears a mask the exposure will be reduced slightly is absurd if everyone is wearing masks that are 98% INEFFECTIVE to begin with. Ask yourself: how do the materials in my mask rate? For all you know, you may be wearing the worst of the worst, and so too all your neighbors.

From the foregoing alone it can easily be seen how it can be the case that COVID is spreading despite people wearing masks. People think they are protective, when they are not. Since they are not, COVID spreads. Simple. But it is worse than that.

The fact that cloth masks are not protective appears to be an open secret among scientists.

In a recent piece, FEATURED IN THE NEW YORK TIMES, but published in the New England Journal of Medicine on Oct. 29, 2020, the scientists literally call for universal masking because… wait for it… ***people wearing such masks are more likely to get COVID.***

So here we have a very large segment of the population believing masks will prevent people from getting COVID when in fact we have examples where not only will most masks do no such thing, but in fact universal use of them, observationally speaking, veritably ENSURES people get COVID.

They write:

> "The typical rate of asymptomatic infection with SARS-COV-2 was estimated to be 40% by the CDC in mid-July, but asymptomatic **infection rates are reported to be higher than 80% in settings with universal facial masking**, which provides observational evidence for this hypothesis."

This appears to be a reference to "an outbreak on a closed Argentinian cruise ship […] where passengers were provided with surgical masks and staff with N95 masks, the rate of asymptomatic infection was 81%" … "compared with 20% in earlier cruise ship outbreaks without universal masking." !!!!

They give several other examples. You may ask yourself what kind of monsters these scientists must be. They appear to know that, contrary to some of their own remarks, 'masks don't work.' But they aren't monsters, I think. They attempt to redeem their position by arguing that the masks increase the chance that the virus is transmitted in smaller amounts, resulting in less severe infections, and thus increase 'herd immunity' with fewer complications. (Normally, invoking 'herd immunity' can get you beaten to an inch of your life, but you can invoke it so long as you endorse every restrictive measure known to man while invoking it.) Be that as it may, the whole premise of their argument depends on masks *not working.*

Besides the simple fact that the materials under discussion can't compete against viruses, especially aerosolized, and people presume too much protection when wearing them and therefore perhaps act 'irresponsibly,' are there any other reasons to help us understand why universal masking fails?

Many of the studies tell us why, but many

people don't want to listen. I am speaking, I hope, to people who do want to listen.

How do we explain such strange results, where infection rates are *higher* in "settings with universal facial masking"?

First of all, invoking 'masks' and discussing whether or not they 'work' is awash in equivocations. An 'equivocation' is when the same word is used to mean different things. It is a logical fallacy when it is done at the same time, without being clear about the differences. It is a little shocking that our public health minders refuse to be clear about these differences, but that is a different essay.

First, 'masks.' N95s (technically, respirators) are indeed effective (95%) if properly fit to the face and handled correctly, mindful of their limitations. But compulsory masking isn't requiring everyone to wear N95s, are they? Then you have surgical masks (2% to 98% effective, see above), and then finally, 'homemade' varieties of masks made with cloth and what not.

As for whether or not they 'work,' the studies have, to this point, largely been confined to trained medical staffers, such as the Vietnam study ("A cluster randomised trial of cloth masks compared with medical masks in healthcare workers" 2015). Most studies do not attempt to measure the effectiveness of widespread masking in the wider public, largely because the wider public has not been masked at a scale that could be studied.

The Vietnam study referenced above sheds further light on this dimension.

Here is what it concludes about the use of *cloth* masks, as worn by **trained health care workers**:

> This study is **the first** RCT [randomised clinical trial] of cloth masks, and the results caution against the use of cloth masks. This is an important finding to inform occupational health and safety. Moisture retention, reuse of cloth masks and poor filtration **may result in increased risk of infection**. Further research is needed … However, as a precautionary measure, cloth masks **should not** be recommended for HCWs, particularly in high-risks situations...

Emphasis added.

The study emphasizes the fact that this is the FIRST such study… and it was only published in 2015.

While they single out cloth masks, what were the results for the 'medical' masks?

Well, out of the 569 participants who wore cloth masks, 31 were still diagnosed with a 'laboratory-confirmed virus.' Out of the 580 participants who wore 'medical masks'19 were diagnosed in the lab with a virus. We can quibble over whether or not *either* 'worked' when A., the difference between the two groups is only 12 individuals and B., the control group—which still wore masks!—had 18. The spread for clinical diagnosis was a bit higher, but not by much (medical = 28, cloth = 43, control = 32). It is a statistically significant difference, but not, to my eye, a very marked difference.

That is to say, if my goal was to keep myself from getting a virus, I would not rely on either a cloth mask, *or* a medical mask.

That said, what they say about the cloth masks after performing their analysis is quite disturbing, in light of the fact that all of our mask mandates are satisfied merely by wearing cloth masks:

> The study suggests medical masks **may** be protective, but the magnitude of differences raises the possibility that **cloth masks cause an increase in infection risk in HCWs.**

Emphasis added.

Allow me to repeat:

[it is possible] cloth masks cause an increase in infection risk in HCWs

Another comprehensive study of studies, published in May of 2020, ("Nonpharmaceutical Measures for Pandemic Influenza in Nonhealthcare Settings—Personal Protective and Environmental Measures") is positively frightening in its implications, revealing in the first place the near malpractice of our health care officials and politicians of declaring that what they are doing is based on 'science', and in the second place, laying bare the fact that our best measures have very little success at preventing the spread of flu-like diseases.

It was easiest just to share the chart summarizing the results of the meta-study. The highlights are mine.

Table 1. Summary of literature searches for systematic review on personal and environmental nonpharmaceutical interventions for pandemic influenza*

Types of interventions	No. studies identified	Study designs included†	Main findings
Hand hygiene	12	RCT	The evidence from RCTs suggested that hand hygiene interventions do not have a substantial effect on influenza transmission.
Respiratory etiquette	0	NA	We did not identify research evaluating the effectiveness of respiratory etiquette on influenza transmission.
Face masks	10	RCT	The evidence from RCTs suggested that the use of face masks either by infected persons or by uninfected persons does not have a substantial effect on influenza transmission.
Surface and object cleaning	3	RCT, observational studies	There was a limited amount of evidence suggesting that surface and object cleaning does not have a substantial effect on influenza transmission.

*NA, not available; RCT randomized controlled trial.

†In these systematic reviews, we prioritized RCTs, and only considered observational studies if there were a small number of RCTs. Our rationale was that with evidence from a larger number of RCTs, additional evidence from observational studies would be unlikely to change overall conclusions.

I would like to once again highlight the date, as I believe chronology is important here. This meta-study was from May 2020. At that time, they could only identify 10 studies on masks, and the general consensus of these studies were that 'masks' did not 'work.' It would have been this scant pool of studies which our public health professionals, such as the surgeon general and Herr Fauci had to go off of. This raises serious questions about their integrity as they then shifted to calling for mask mandates. On what basis could they possibly have made these calls?

Nonetheless, their calls were heeded, and what amounted to an experiment on humans without their consent, on a mass scale, henceforth followed. (For background, start with the Nuremberg Code and work your way forward.) We are beginning to see the results of this experiment, sometimes released to us in the form of a study, rather than anecdote.

The CDC itself, in data announced back in July but published in September, determined that face masking showing little success in preventing the spread of COVID.

Out of the 314 people who participated in the study (154 COVID positive, 160 COVID negative), the vast majority reported "ALWAYS" wearing a mask. 226. Another 50 reported ‘often’ wearing a mask. The differences between the two groups was miniscule, but not my point. **130 of the 154 fell ill whilst ‘often’ or ‘always’ wearing a mask.**

To rebut the obvious implications of this, comments like “well, they must have interacted with people not wearing a mask” are said. But, as with the Marquette study I referenced at the beginning, in actuality, overall compliance was quite high. In the COVID-negative group, 141 out of the 160 reported ‘often’ or ‘always’ wearing their masks. If they are ones who had gone to a restaurant, they were asked if others were also complying: 41% said that everyone around them was complying almost all the time, 39.7% said that half/most were complying. Only 19% said that no one was complying. Since the CDC report did not have mask efficacy in view with its report, we cannot put too much weight on this. But as a snapshot, it admits a largely compliant population. In the CDC sample, 72% reported “ALWAYS” wearing the mask.

In mid-July New York Times article, which discussed the results of an investigation spanning a whopping 250,000 people, they asserted:

> Despite these variations, and despite the flare-ups over the issue that pepper social media, the rates of self-reported mask use in the United States are high. **Several national surveys in recent weeks have found that around 80 percent of Americans say they wear masks frequently or always when they expect to be within six feet of other people.** That number falls short of the sort of universal masking many public health officials have asked for, but it is higher than the rates of mask use in several other countries, including Canada, Finland and Denmark, according to a recent survey from YouGov.

Emphasis added.

It is time to stop with the cop-out rebuttal that the problem is non-compliance. In fact, let's just translate it into its real meaning. People who blame the spread of COVID on non-compliance are really saying, "If only those selfish bastards would wear their masks we wouldn't be in this mess." This is not an argument from evidence. The evidence is that compliance was relatively high and remains relatively high. It is an argument from arrogance. STOP IT.

Moving on.

The now infamous Danish study ("Effectiveness of Adding a Mask Recommendation to Other Public Health Measures to Prevent SARS-CoV-2 Infection in Danish Mask Wearers") that came out a few weeks ago was one of the first to really start exploring the results of wearing masks in the wider community rather than just health care professionals. I'll spare you the agony and jump right to the conclusion:

> The recommendation to wear **surgical masks** to supplement other public health measures **did not** reduce the SARS-CoV-2 infection rate among wearers by more than 50% in a community with modest infection rates, some degree of social distancing, and uncommon general mask use. The data were compatible with lesser degrees of self-protection.

Emphasis added.

This was from Denmark in April and May of 2020, the peak of the COVID nightmare around the world for most countries. (As of this writing, I did not research whether or not

Denmark itself was experiencing a peak.)

In the spirit of keeping our kinds of 'masks' straight, we notice that they specifically measured were surgical masks, not cloth masks. Since surgical/medical masks are modestly more effective than cloth masks (see discussion above, from the Vietnam study), we can only imagine how much less cloth masks would 'work' in the wider community.

It does specify that there was 'uncommon general mask use' so there is still some small sliver of hope for the pro-muzzlers to cling to, lurking to their old standby retort that 'if only EVERYONE was wearing their mask!' That is why I have tackled that first, by showing that even in largely compliant populations, COVID is still spreading… nay, SURGING! If you can't blame the 'selfish bastards' because the evidence leans away from that, you need to begin exploring other possibilities.

Shortly after the Danish study was released, we had a remarkable report released which I would be remiss if I did not mention here. This is the Nov. 19, 2020 "SARS-COV-2 Transmission among Marine Recruits during Quarantine."

Before we evaluate the findings of this

study, we need to talk about yet another equivocation that is prevalent, and that is the equivocation of the word 'works.' You know, in the question, "do masks 'work'?"

As described above, first of all we need to ask what *kinds* of masks, and *what* do we hope to achieve with them? Even in many of these studies, it is not often specified what kind of mask is in view. (I have tried to limit myself to the ones where it *is* specified in this essay.) By 'work' do we mean, "will stop large droplets"? or do we mean "filter out viruses that are very small?"

And in what *context?* A surgeon standing relatively stationary over a patient wearing a surgical mask is a trained individual performing a very specific task. I can assure you, if the person he was operating on had ebola, he would not be satisfied only wearing a surgical mask! Would anyone like to wager money on this?

What about running, jumping, sweating, fidgeting, and other such 'contexts'? Athletes are being compelled to wear masks of various sorts. Unlike surgeons, they aren't just standing there! The movement invariably means adjusting and re-adjusting their face covering, regardless of what kind of mask it is. Will a mask 'work' in this context, where it is being handled frequently to get it right on the face, people are breathing heavily through it and on it, and sweat is pouring over it? What do you think happens to the efficacy of a face mask if it is wet? Do you assume it will keep working? Based on what? There are no studies measuring the efficacy of any kind of mask by soccer players competing in the rain. But that doesn't stop our 'intelligentsia' from requiring soccer players to wear masks, even if it is raining!

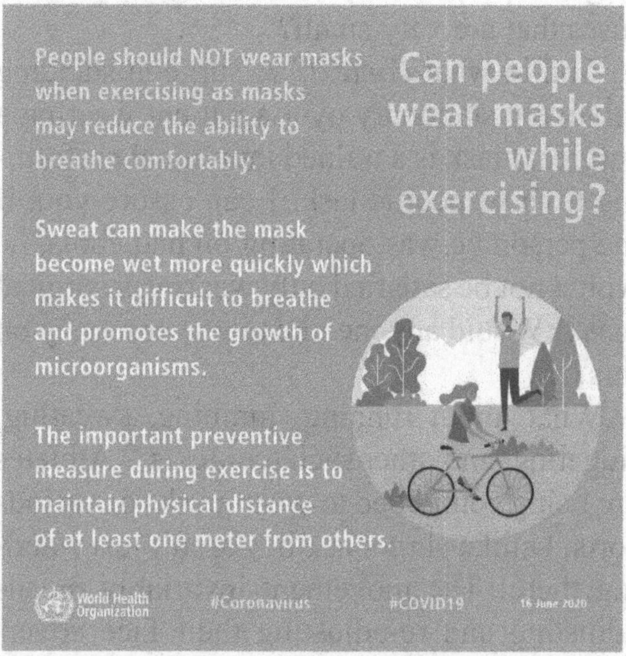

Can people wear masks while exercising?
People should NOT wear masks when exercising as masks may reduce the ability to breathe comfortably.
Sweat can make the mask become wet more quickly which makes it difficult to breathe and promotes the growth of microorganisms.
The important preventive measure during exercise is to maintain physical distance of at least one meter from others.
World Health Organization
#Coronavirus
#COVID19

Don't misunderstand me. I don't have great faith in the WHO either. But even a broken clock is right twice a day.

Will a mask 'work' if you wear it 8 hours straight in a context which avoids either extreme (moving rapidly vs standing stationary)? That is, shopping in a mall and then going to a big box store and finally a grocery store? The evidence says "Hell no!" regardless of context, but *why not?* How about for 8 hours, getting in and out of cars, going up and down stairs, pushing carts, handling goods which won't be sanitized before the next person grabs, them, scratching your nose—first from the outside, and then when you really can't get the itch, then on the inside, with your gloveless finger, which you then put on the credit card machine—and so on.

Will your mask work in *that* context?

?

The study I referenced earlier in this essay ("Simple Respiratory Protection") determined that cloth masks "had 40-90% instantaneous penetration levels" but this was in a laboratory setting, simulating the wearing of masks and using machines to blow things into and through them. I hope I don't have to explain to the reader that robots are not walking around with cloth stretched over their orifices hoping to protect themselves from nozzles shooting aerosols at them. No, we are being asked… nay, told… to *live* with these face coverings.

There are no studies which measure whether or not these measures 'work' in *that* context. The Danish one is one of the first ones to make the attempt, and it was only released a few weeks ago, months after our nanny do-gooders began making us wear masks. Not on the basis of science, as I have shown, so I guess just for the hell of it.

I said all of that to set up my remarks about the Marines.

Outside of the wet dreams of our public health officials and certain governors, it is practically speaking impossible to get 100% compliance with 100% of all measures they wish to mandate. The intricate details of the daily life of 350,000,000 is beyond the reach of anyone but God himself. (Note: you are NOT God.)

You can't even get 100% compliance with 100% of all measures in a 100% captive environment. However, no one is going to get closer than the US Marines. In a remarkable study which demanded that new recruits quarantine 14 days before arrival, upon which a number of them were quarantined *even more*, they discovered that at the end of the study's 14 days, soldiers *not* subjected to these extra-stringent measures tested positive for COVID *less than* those who were subjected to extra-stringent measures!

26 nonparticipants out of 1,554 tested positive at the end of 14 days (1.7%) whereas 51 of the 1,848 'participants' tested positive (2.8%).

There are a number of really remarkable aspects of this study, not least of which is the fact that there were nearly double the number of COVID cases where every quarantine measure conceivable—including masking—was inflicted, as opposed to those who weren't. This appears to be indirect corroboration of the fact that *all* these measures ***increase*** infection rates, rather than decrease them!

This is not the general public. Six Marine instructors for each platoon worked 8 hour shifts to enforce the quarantine measures. There is not the tiniest sliver left of the argument that the reason why people got COVID is because of non-compliance. This is a study where compliance was extraordinarily high, well beyond what is possible in the general public.

To get a full taste, one really ought to read the whole thing. Here is a long excerpt, with emphasis added:

> To reduce the risk of introducing SARS-CoV-2 into basic training at Marine Corps Recruit Depot, Parris Island, in South Carolina, the Marine **Corps established a 14-day supervised quarantine period at a college campus used exclusively for this purpose. Potential recruits were instructed to quarantine at home for 2 weeks immediately before they traveled to campus.** At the end of the second, supervised quarantine on campus, all recruits were required to have a negative qPCR result before they could enter Parris Island. Recruits were asked to participate in the COVID-19 Health Action Response for Marines (CHARM) study, which included weekly qPCR testing and blood sampling for IgG antibody assessment.
>
> […]

During the supervised quarantine, public health measures were enforced to suppress SARS-CoV-2 transmission. **All recruits wore double-layered cloth masks at all times indoors and outdoors, except when sleeping or eating**; practiced social distancing of **at least 6 feet**; were not allowed to leave campus; **did not have access to personal electronics and other items that might contribute to surface transmission; and routinely washed their hands.** They slept in double-occupancy rooms with sinks, ate in shared dining facilities, and used shared bathrooms. All recruits cleaned their rooms daily, sanitized bathrooms after each use with bleach wipes, and ate preplated meals in a dining hall that was cleaned with bleach after each platoon had eaten. Most instruction and exercises were conducted outdoors. **All movement of recruits was supervised**, and unidirectional flow was implemented, with designated building entry and exit points to minimize contact among persons. All recruits, regardless of participation in the study, underwent daily temperature and symptom screening. **Six instructors who were assigned to each platoon worked in 8-hour shifts and enforced the quarantine measures.**

[...] Instructors were also restricted to campus, were required to wear masks, were provided with preplated meals, and underwent daily temperature checks and symptom screening. Instructors who were assigned to a platoon in which a positive case was diagnosed underwent rapid qPCR testing for SARS-CoV-2, and, if the result was positive, the instructor was removed from duty. Recruits and instructors were prohibited from interacting with campus support staff, such as janitorial and food-service personnel. After each class completed quarantine, a deep bleach cleaning of surfaces was performed in the bathrooms, showers, bedrooms, and hallways in the dormitories, and the dormitory remained unoccupied for at least 72 hours before reoccupancy.

And yet, after 30 days of quarantine, half of which was enforced by one of the world's most pre-eminent military services, 77 people still tested positive for COVID. More than half of these were treated to extra-extra precautions, and almost twice as many of *them* got COVID as those not subjected to those extra-extra precautions.

Not only does that spell doom for the idea that compulsory masking 'works' it strongly suggests that nothing short of killing people, removing all possible way for the virus to spread from person to person (because they are all dead), will prevent COVID from spreading. I assume the reader believes that option should be off the table. Personally, I think having 8 Marine instructors for every 'platoon' of the general citizenry monitoring our every move should be off the table, too, as even with that, we see the measures did not succeed in fully suppressing the virus. (A virus, I'd add, is 99%+ survivable by almost the entire population.)

From the foregoing it should be evident that if one is truly concerned about protecting one's self from COVID, there really are only a few things that you can do, and these are things you must do for yourself. Forcing other people to engage in activities or precluding them from doing so is *not* going to be helpful. This will only create a false sense of security and probably lead you to do something that, despite your good intentions, actually results in infecting yourself or others.

Obviously, quarantining yourself for an extended period of time—forever, I reckon—is your only sure bet. But any and every potential human interaction, including having items mailed to you, and other distant connections, contains risk. That said, I know of no one who objects to individuals or families locking themselves away indefinitely. The problem is when they wish to inflict on others what they only have a right to inflict on themselves.

Listen carefully, as I'm going to now going to tell you how you really can maximize your protection.

If one does dare to step outside and interact with humanity, it must be recognized that cloth masks **cannot** be relied on. I'm not talking here about some kind of statistical gambit where one reasons that the small protection one has multiplied by the small protection other people have theoretically results in a somewhat improved protection for everyone. I'm talking about YOU, as an individual.

Let's say, for example, you are in a known vulnerable sub-group. Over eighty with a heart condition, maybe, and very concerned that COVID would be the death of you. You would be an absolute fool, now that you are aware of what I've just shared, to entrust yourself to a cloth mask. Only a slightly less foolish fool to entrust yourself to a medical mask.

The masks with the best protection in any reliable sense are the N95s. But YOU have got to wear them correctly. YOU have to make sure they are properly fit. YOU have to make sure that you handle them correctly. No one can make YOU do these things.

But here is the kicker: You must wear gloves, as well. And eye protection. And you cannot scratch your nose from the inside of the N95. Then you have to properly remove the items so as to not contaminate yourself in the process. YOU must do all of these things, or else all of your gear is useless.

It is critical that you understand this. Insofar as any studies have demonstrated the plausibility that masks (of any sort) 'work,' the argument is that they 'work' because (presumably) the chief source of the spread are the large droplets coming from your mouth. Being larger droplets, they will have a higher viral load, making infection more likely and more acute if you are the hapless chap on the receiving end of spittle flinging through the air. But take a moment to think through the mechanics of what is assumed in this scenario:

A person with COVID sends a mini-goober of death hurtling through the air. No worries, you are protected, because it lands on your mask, and does not get through! The crowd cheers! Then, probably not two minutes after this, you put your hand on the mask right where the saliva got caught 'effectively' by your mask.

Then, your fingers, which have now been dipped in a droplet of spit brimming over with COVID like a paint brush dipped into paint, now begins touching things... such as your own nose. Yea, sure, you tried to scratch your itch from outside the mask, but it just didn't take. So, against your better judgement, you slip that 'paint brush' between the mask and your face and give your nose a proper scratch. If you've ever painted, you understand precisely why I give this analogy.

An hour later, you get a bit drowsy, and, after adjusting your mask countless times between the arrival of the rona-bomb on your mask and that moment, you rub your eyes.

If you ever see a study which shows that masks 'work,' especially in the general public, you can be confident that it does not take into account the real-life experience of wearing masks for hours and hours on end. And of course, we are ignoring for this exercise the reality that certain masks, like cloth ones, may indeed stop a large droplet, but other stuff is just going to fly through it.

Remember that thing about having a 'false sense of security'?

So, if you're going to wear a mask, wear the N95s and wear them right! Along with all the other gear.

It is critical that another thing be pointed out: improving your overall health is really the number 1 thing that you can do, as we know that it's the people with underlying conditions that are the most vulnerable. But even that doesn't do the truth justice: people without underlying conditions are almost completely safe. Almost.

The only 'masks' that 'work' are the N95, but only if properly fitted, properly donned and removed, and so on. But viruses are not spread only via the mouth and nose. The eyes are also a vulnerability.

Guess what? If YOU take these precautions, it won't matter what other people do (assuming they aren't tackling you or something like that) because you will have obtained about the most protection that you can get.

But remember… even this did not spare 2.7% of the Marines. (Granted, while the Marines inflicted every restriction known to man with near 100% compliance obtained, the masks were only double-layered cloth ones.)

So, I guess you need to decide: you can either get busy living, or you can get busy dying. But this is in YOUR hands. You don't need anyone else to do anything else. Maybe if people started actually minding their own business, COVID will die away fairly quickly.

I know what you're thinking.

"Waitaminute. Why would it die away fairly quickly?"

Because you have to flip it all around.

If universal masking, especially if cloth masks are deemed perfectly satisfactory for fulfilling our mask mandates, potentially increases the risk of infection, *why* is that the case? Because in the general population, containing mostly untrained individuals, LIVING with a mask on your face for hours and hours on end means constantly touching your face, your facemask, and so on.

I was recently in a meeting where every person in the room was wearing a mask. I watched as every single person in that room touched their mask, removed it to talk, touched their face without the mask on, put the mask back on, fidgeted with it some more, so on and so forth. Hey, I'm not blaming them, I was doing the same thing! (I just wasn't deluded into thinking my cloth mask protected me). These were smart people who really thought they were doing the right thing. The 'elite,' as it were. How often do you think the commoners are touching their face and face mask all the time?

You see it now, right?

If you are NOT wearing a mask, the number of times your hands go to the face to adjust the face mask is radically reduced. It isn't just the fact that your breath gets through these masks, or around, or is redirected behind you, but the fact that they are constantly handled, that is the problem. And it is IMPOSSIBLE to have even a slightly active lifestyle without constantly handling your facemask.

Remember, the surgeon we hear constantly invoked is not just wearing a mask. He is wearing gloves. He is trained on how to don them and remove them. More to the point, he's not doing jumping jacks. He's pretty much fixed in place. It is an entirely unique context which does not describe how the rest of us live our lives, most of the time.

In conclusion, it really shouldn't be any surprise that so many studies have revealed that face masking is unlikely to work in the general public. The only really surprising thing is that anyone needed a study to tell them what they could have figured out themselves just watching humans going about their daily business… or even watched themselves do so.

Bottom line: if anything, universal masking is leaving vulnerable people vulnerable. It is a failed policy and needs to be abandoned by people of integrity IMMEDIATELY.

Bottom-bottom line: if you are concerned about your own health, settle for nothing less than N95s, goggles, and disposable gloves, which you have taken the time to learn how to handle appropriately, and disciplined yourself to apply what you have learned.

https://www.marquette.edu/news-center/2020/marquette-researchers-find-90-percent-of-wisconsin-residents-in-compliance-with-state-mask-mandate.php

https://twitter.com/surgeon_general/status/1233725785283932160?lang=en

https://www.nytimes.com/interactive/2020/07/17/upshot/coronavirus-face-mask-map.html

https://www.facebook.com/WHO/photos/a.167668209945237/3245900815455279/?type=3

https://www.msn.com/en-us/health/medical/the-who-says-masks-shouldnt-be-worn-during-intense-physical-activity-contradicting-other-advice/ar-BB1bzj6f?ocid=msedgntp

https://www.nytimes.com/2020/09/08/health/covid-masks-immunity.html?smid=tw-nythealth&smtyp=cur

I'm making you look up the studies yourself. I provided the names and years of each study in the body of the text. Seeing people engage in critical thinking and independent research is what we desperately need right now, and I shall not deprive the reader of the opportunity to exercise these skills.

https://www.manhattanmedicalnews.com/news-letter/2020/august/researchers-find-84-percent-of-residents-in-compliance-with-face-mask-mandate.htm

https://twitter.com/sugargeneuk/status/1234778578311760?lang=en

https://www.nytimes.com/interactive/2020/07/14/business/coronavirus-face-mask-map.html

https://www.facebook.com/WHO/photos/a.167668209945237/2458158154522?type=3

https://www.msn.com/en-us/health/medical/health-experts-masks-shouldnt-be-common-use-in-general-public/ar-BB10GCdi?ocid=msedgntp

https://www.nytimes.com/2020/07/07/health/covid-masks-immunity.html?smid=tw-nytimes&smtyp=cur

I'm asking you look up the studies yourself. I provided the names and years of each study in the body of the text. Seeing people engage in critical thinking and independent research is what we desperately need right now, and I shall not deprive the reader of the opportunity to exercise these skills.

Post Script

Finally, without getting into it too much, I feel that I need to at least mention something that arose out of those early days in late Feb and March when our numerous luminaries told us to STOP BUYING MASKS. Have you ever wondered why it is that they had to say that? I mean, given the current resistance against universal masking right now, don't you find it the least bit surprising that at the beginning, everyone and their mother was eager to acquire and wear them? Was there an edict from the king in January that told everyone to go out and buy them, and then suddenly the lords and ladies who rule us decided on a course change? No, this did not happen.

What happened was that 350,000,000 people decided, on their own estimation and evaluation of the situation, what their best course of action was and then they pursued it. You didn't have to tell them to buy and wear masks, because if, as a general rule, people are idiots (as a friend of mine who a public health official recently told me), they are still self-interested enough not to want to kill themselves. We know this was the case, because the elites had to come out strongly and tell them, not merely that they should STOP

BUYING MASKS, they ALSO SAID… wait for it… MASKS DON'T WORK.

It was only by telling people that MASKS DON'T WORK that they were able to convince people to stop buying them, because people reasoned to themselves that there was no point in buying something that didn't work.

The dirty little secret is that you generally don't need to tell people what is good for them and more often than not you don't have to *command* them to do what is good for them. Miraculously, people find out what is good for them and do it on their own without being compelled to do so. Can you believe it? No, it's true. There are no laws commanding people to eat, or sleep, for example. As stupid as they are (according to public health officials), people can figure out quite a bit on their own.

Which means that if people are no longer wearing masks or feeling amenable to complying with lock down measures anymore, it could be because they are selfish asshats (one theory) or… or… *the evidence itself simply does not warrant such measures.* For, if it did, you wouldn't have to force them to take those measures. See how it works?

Eight months later, give or take, we have a

good handle on what the 'novel' coronavirus is all about. Even if it was deliberately created or released from a Wuhan lab, there doesn't appear to be another shoe to drop. We know that the vast majority of people who get COVID will not even have any symptoms at all, or if they do, they will be so mild it could be mistaken for just feeling a bit run down. We know who the vulnerable people are, and we know that for the rest of us the survivability rate is better than 99% and even for the vulnerable, it is still around that number.

Vulnerable people should indeed be taking precautions. Hopefully after reading my essay they will take even better precautions. On the other hand, going forward in the future, when we start caring about the flu again, these may wish to remember what really works and what really does not.

Bossing around your fellow man, to the tune of millions of them, is not an option which is going to go over well in the long term. That is to say, if you push tens of millions too far, you may discover to your great displeasure that the asymptomatic spread of an eminently survivable disease is the least of your concerns. Or, you may stumble across another lesson writ large in history related to the wisdom (or complete lack thereof) of giving one or two people or an elite clutch of them the decision-making power over the most minute daily affairs of 350,000,000 people. If you don't get my gist, you may start with Orwell's *Animal Farm*, and work your way from there.

It would be better if we did not encounter either of those eventualities, but the conduct of our elites and the sheeple to this point seem to suggest that we won't be happy until we definitely conclude with one or the other. If, per chance, we avoid either, there is still the other possible outcome: a virus that actually is absolutely lethal, which definitively is a bioweapon or what have you, lands on our shores, and nobody believes it because we've been fed one lie after another about a virus which was rendered a veritable "yawn" (as compared to all other threats to our well-being which we are all aware of), and no longer trust anything that is said.

Wouldn't that be unfortunate?

www.ingramcontent.com/pod-product-compliance
Lightning Source LLC
Chambersburg PA
CBHW011803040426
42450CB00017B/3452
* 9 7 8 1 6 4 5 9 4 0 5 3 1 *